Genetically Modified Foods vs. Sustainability

By Bruno McGrath

Copyright © 2012 Bruno McGrath & Pandora Poikilos

All rights reserved. Except for use in any review, the reproduction or utilization of this work in whole or in part in any form by any electronic, mechanical or other means, now known or hereafter invented, including xerography, photocopying and recording, or in any information storage or retrieval system is forbidden.

ISBN-13: 978-1484956472
ISBN-10: 1484956478

CONTENTS

Genetically Modified Foods vs. Sustainability
- 1.1 Introduction
- 1.2 Commercial Interests
- 1.3 Capitalism vs. Agriculture
- 1.4 Land Management
- 1.5 Population Control
- 1.6 Permaculture
- 1.7 Healthy Eating
- 1.8 Knowledge is Power
- 1.9 Combined Efforts
- 1.10 Conclusion

Opinion Poll - But What Are You Eating

Bibliography

1.1 Introduction

In an age of no social media and lack of transparency, more than 20 million gallons of herbicide were sprayed throughout South Vietnam, Laos and Cambodia between 1962 and 1971. The target? Guerrillas who would be forced to come out in the open instead of hiding in the jungle. The objective? To ensure the population would flee to areas dominated by the US. The effect? More than 5 million people including US soldiers were exposed to this herbicide otherwise known as Agent Orange.

Its effects have said to be present to this day with people in certain areas prone to skin diseases, birth defects and a string of genetic diseases. The American public was not made aware of this issue until after 1965 by which time most of the damage had been done. Lawsuits were eventually brought against the companies that were involved and although financial settlements were made, denial continues to reign. The blame shifts at every turn with no single party taking responsibility for the outcome of Agent Orange.

The company that manufactured the herbicide? Monsanto. Over the years, it has made a strong attempt at disconnecting itself from Agent Orange, a task far easier said than done. It now markets itself as a seed and agricultural company but continues to court controversy. As with the Agent Orange lawsuits, Monsanto has been able to shield itself from any permanent damage despite public outcry at its products and business practices.

More recently, Monsanto has dominated the American food market with its genetically modified seeds. It continues to stress that after significant research and development, this is the best way to ensure sustainability. Can genetically modified produce effect sustainability and increase food supply? Of course it can. But it is not the best way and it is definitely not the only way.

First and foremost, the amount of time that has been devoted to research of genetically modified produce raises many concerns. For centuries, farmers have been harvesting crop using traditional methods. Negative side effects, if any, have only occurred when human error is involved. Hence, how many decades have genetically modified produce been dissected to guarantee there are no or minimal side effects? Monsanto provides a different answer from what is documented but either way, no official source is able to guarantee safety of genetically modified produce.

More importantly, and this is a question that most consumers should start asking themselves, is quantity more important than quality? Are general consumers being given all the facts they need before they choose what is good for them? There are too many unanswered questions where genetically modified produce is concerned and the exact motivations of its existence appear to be more questionable than beneficial.

1.2 Commercial Interests

The media makes great effort to shed a bleak look at the future, often stressing that the world will run out of food in a few years and that people in highly populated areas will be the first to suffer. Essentially, this is where sustainability becomes a push and pull topic and appears as if it is always another country that is facing the difficulties of sustainable living.

This portrayal also makes it seem that sustainability is a corporate problem. In other words, it is the large corporations that should worry about where food comes from and this should not concern the public. Hence, the increased levels of commercial interests in sustainability and the issue of sustainability are no longer viewed as a necessity to healthy living but as a money-making effort for the future.

For instance, Somalia's current and past situation needs no introduction. For more than two decades it has been used as the best example of a failed and starving state. It has been riddled with one problem after another. If Mother Nature does not tear it apart, it is shredded to pieces by the Al-Shabaab who claim their actions are necessary to protect their people from the West. A picture speaks a thousand words and Somalia has had too many pictures of malnutrition, women dying at childbirth, starvation and poverty. There are no banks. Development is non-existent. Luxury is when someone is able to survive on $60 a month.

The London Conference 2012 was held in February 2012 and more than 40 countries pledged financial aid for the country.

Is there truly no commercial interest in this financial aid? That remains to be seen. Somalia may be riddled with non-development but it has vast land that can be cultivated for agriculture. So when countries take 20 years to pledge aid, which problem are they actually solving and whose commercial interests are being protected? The starvation from the past or sustainability for the future?

On the other hand is commercial interest in sustainability entirely a bad thing? When applied in moderation, it isn't. In actual fact, it is one of the best ways to raise consumer awareness about the issue. While Monsanto has devoted time and energy to raising awareness about genetically modified produce, other companies such as Coca Cola and Waitrose have taken a different route in doing their part to ensure sustainable living.

With more than 10 million coolers and vending machines in place, Coca Cola announced in 2009 that it had identified a natural refrigerant that would be replacing its hydrofluorocarbon (HFC) coolers. It is expected that the company will phase out its HFC coolers by 2015, and this effort is equal to taking at least 11 millions cars off the road per year. To date, the company claims that it is on track to reaching this goal and Greenpeace supports this claim.

Waitrose has made a conscious effort to inform its consumers about what they are eating. It has so far taken a firm stand in stating that no genetically modified produce will be sold by the company or by its suppliers. In a campaign known as "The Waitrose Way" the company continues to highlight its method of food sourcing, its role in championing British food suppliers and its overall efforts to ensure its consumers treated to a healthy lifestyle.

1.3 Capitalism vs. Agriculture

How does one company stay unscathed from continual blazing controversy? From its production of herbicide to now a growing seed giant, Monsanto is adamant that their efforts are for a better future for all mankind. In 1980, there were no official records of genetically modified seeds ever being grown or researched in the United States. In 2007, more than 142 million acres were planted in the United States and more than 280 million across the globe. Monsanto itself now accounts for at least 90 per cent of the production of soybean in the United States.

Hence, the most fuelling question of all. How can a product that has not been tested on the lifespan of a human being be deemed safe? Monsanto has been asked this question many times before, one it chooses to conveniently ignore and cushion with its profits. The company claims that the monopoly it holds offers better jobs and lifestyles for medium-sized agricultural companies and family farmers.

But the feedback from farmers who have signed with Monsanto tells a different story. Those who have been willing to speak against the giant claim that the long list of farmers who have signed up with Monsanto were either arm twisted into an agreement with the company or were not fully aware of what they were getting themselves into. Up to 2007, Monsanto has taken at least 112 farmers throughout the United States to court.

Farmers have found themselves being followed, video taped and probed by private investigators. Monsanto claims these efforts are necessary to protect its patents and to ensure that the farmers they are working with abide by the agreements the company has signed with them. But are agreements and patents the way forward for the agricultural sector? If sustainability is truly the core of Monsanto's genetically modified produce, should it not be available to everyone?

Most farmers who are taken to court by Monsanto eventually give in and pay a settlement. They know that their medium-sized plots of land and produce cannot compete with a company that has unlimited resources. How it retains so much power is a question that may be unanswered for decades to come. For instance, Monsanto was recently sued by 83 plaintiffs who represented more than 300,000 organic farmers. On 31st January 2012, opening arguments were heard and a court date was set. Triumph for the farmers was short-lived as Monsanto appealed and the case was dismissed on 29th February 2012. Will it be the last time Monsanto is taken to court, probably not.

Singer and Farm Aid activist, Willie Nelson, who is one of the millions who are against Monsanto's tactics and produces. He stressed that the corporate control of the food system has been a major contributing factor to the destruction of the country's soil. Would sustainability be achievable without capitalism? It might be a difficult venture especially on a global scale. But sustainability can definitely thrive without a monopoly.

An opinion poll – But What Are You Eating – was conducted in February 2012 to gather feedback on consumer awareness about genetically modified produce. A respondent from the Philippines stated that while the farmers in his country were either only just above the poverty line or middle-class and had never heard of genetically modified produce. Of course, this meant that their produce was almost fresh and this ignorance towards genetically modified produce was a blessing in disguise.

1.4 Land Management

Between climate issues, an increasing world population, economic downturns and stagnant employment rates, one of the major concerns most countries face is land management. What is the ratio of land for buildings versus sustainable growth for agriculture?

Contrary to popular belief, land management doesn't affect rural areas as much as it affects urban areas of a country. Higher population means more buildings, which in turn mean more pollution and a higher use of resources without the complete assurance of a sustainable lifestyle.

Additionally, countries such as Australia, Japan and some parts of Eastern Europe have been having difficulty in maintaining their crops after being hit by natural disasters. Australia is a major exporter of sugar and had many of its sugarcane fields destroyed by major flooding, while the 2011 earthquake in Japan resulted in a nuclear scare, which disrupted fishing. The cold wave earlier in 2012 went on to disrupt farming in many Eastern European countries and left a death toll of at least 500 people across Europe.

All of these issues were non-specifically addressed by the United Nations Department of Economic and Social Affairs Division for Sustainable Development in 2009. Six priority areas for governments to implement and enforce were identified. These factors were deemed to be especially crucial to ensure sustainable land management.

The six priority areas are prevention and/or mitigation of land degradation; access to land and security of tenure; critical sectors and issues (such as biodiversity, drylands, rehabilitation of mining areas, wetlands and coastal zones, coral reefs, natural disasters, and rural-urban and land management interactions); access to information and stakeholder participation; international cooperation, including that for capacity-building, information-sharing, and technology transfer; and minerals, metals and rehabilitation of land degraded by mining in the context of sustainable development.

The United Nations Commission on Sustainable Development also concluded that major adjustments were significant and required in agricultural, environmental and macroeconomic policy, at both national and international levels, in developed as well as developing countries, to create the conditions for sustainable agriculture and rural development.

The last time land management issues were reviewed by the UN was in 1995, when it "noted with concern that, even though some progress had been reported, disappointment is widely expressed at the slow progress in moving towards sustainable agriculture and rural development in many countries. Governments were urged to attach high priority to implementing the commitments agreed at the 1996 World Food Summit, especially the call for at least halving the number of undernourished people in the world by the year 2015."

Earth Summit 2012 organised by The United Nations Commission on Sustainable Development is expected to kick off on 20th June 2012 in Rio De Janeiro, Brazil. Its theme this year is "Reaching Sustainable Development Through Knowledge" and is expected to achieve renewed political commitment towards a green economy with sustainable development and poverty eradication. It isn't the first time issues such as reducing disaster risk and building resilience; food security and sustainable culture;

and governance for sustainable development have been discussed at length.

On previous occasions, disagreements have been rampant on the preferred route that countries need to take and it remains to be seen if land management on an international level for sustainable agricultural growth will be an issue that will be dealt with in the immediate future.

1.5 Population Control

China introduced its controversial one-child policy in 1979 and has recently reported that it does not intend to review this policy until 2015 although it made way for some couples to have a second child in March 2011.

Many have argued that this policy is dictatorial, limits personal freedom and can spark an unhealthy economy. While the first two points are debatable, China's economy is anything but unhealthy with even the Eurozone seeking bailout help from its Asian counterpart. Logically, this decision simply means that the population of a country should go hand in hand with a country's growth. If a country does not have enough economic strength and agricultural development, its population should be reduced or at the very least slowed.

How effective will population control be in attaining sustainability? This remains to be an ongoing discovery as the world's population has reached seven billion. It is becoming increasingly important that people in highly populated countries understand the concept of birth control. Whether they choose to practise it is a personal choice but they must be made aware of it and have ready access to it.

In Rift Valley, Kenya in 1985, it was apparent that birth control was a tremendous challenge. The nearest clinic was said to be at least 15 miles away, and its service was spasmodic. In addition, the journey to the clinic would cost the equivalent of nearly $2, a luxury for an average Kenyan woman. On top of it all, it wasn't certain that women who arrived at these clinics were able to see anyone or receive free birth control pills.

"Everyone criticizes the women for having too many children, but if women in the Western world had to travel the distances our women in rural areas are expected to cover to meet an inefficient service, they would be discouraged as well," commented the leader of one women's group.

It would be expected that in more than twenty years, the situation would have improved. It hasn't. Nicholas D. Kristoff from the New York Times made his annual trip across Central Africa in 2009, "the pill, 50 years old this month in the United States, has yet to reach parts of Africa and condoms and other forms of birth control and AIDS prevention are still far too difficult to obtain in some areas."

It isn't just developing countries that need to focus on birth control issues. Birth control should be a choice for any woman for the simple reason that unwanted pregnancies, baby dumping and over flowing orphanages all have a significant impact on sustainability and the long-term development of a country.

Religious and cultural views are often given precedence, and as with the recent issue in the United States, the debate of free birth control options is one that needs to be given more awareness.

In early March 2012, Georgetown Law School student Sandra Fluke testified before the United States congress that birth control had to be included in health insurance plans. A popular radio host, Rush Limbaugh responded to her remarks by saying "What does it say about the college coed … who goes before a congressional committee and essentially says that she must be paid to have sex?" He went on to call her "a slut" and "a prostitute".

While birth control as part of a health insurance plan may not be a viable option for all countries, women cannot be afraid of birth control, in any country be it developed or not. It must always be an available option.

1.6 Permaculture

Otherwise known as permanent agriculture or culture, permaculture is not a new alternative to sustainable living. It is focused on living lightly, and making sure that human activities can be sustained for many generations to come, in harmony with nature. One of the main objectives of permaculture is to give back to nature. In other words, sustainable farming and land cultivation must be carefully planned so soil is regenerative, water conserved and energy saved. Permanence is not about everything staying the same. It is about stability, about deepening soils and cleaner water, thriving communities in self-reliant regions, biodiverse agriculture and social justice, peace and abundance.

The concept originated in 1978 and was the brainchild of David Holmgreen and Bill Mollison. It is currently practised in more than 5 continents and provides sustainable living for a significant number of towns and villages in 20 countries.

Is this a better alternative than genetically modified produce? Some may argue it is not. It is however, an alternative which is the essence of this critical argument. How successful is permaculture in cultivating a sustainable environment? Sceptics argue that permaculture is based on weak economic structure, cannot sustain an urban population and is appreciated by those who wish to embrace a "hippie" or a nomadic lifestyle. The first two are valid arguments while the latter two are misconceptions.

It will be costly and time consuming to apply permaculture on a global scale. In more than three decades, it is still known to benefit smaller communities and is only successful after lengthy training sessions to cultivate a person's skills in ensuring they are able to sustain themselves for housing repair, food supplies and day-to-day necessities. In a nutshell, it teaches one to simplify their lifestyles and be at peace with nature. Does this mean no technology at all? Definitely not. The goal is to use what you need and not waste what you are using.

For example, Scott and Arina Pittman have adopted permaculture for at least two decades. Their home was built to mimic a traditional courtyard house with a massive garden that they use to experiment with plantation. Traditional adobe brick and clay plaster were used for the main structure and walls of the house. Additionally, no toxic materials were used, all wastewater was utilised, electromagnetic fields were limited and passive solar heat was incorporated.

There are different stages of permaculture, some of which can be adopted in any urban home provided enough awareness is raised about it. While the improvements of this practice may not occur immediately, continued practice will result in improved lifestyle and eating habits. Essentially, the benefits of permaculture far outweigh its weaknesses.

A family that can sustain itself for 10 years is far better than a family that relies on the government for aid. Additionally, there still appears to be a lot of scepticism as to how much it can help the environment. Will an increased population that applies permaculture make a difference or is the continual increase in population that needs to be stopped?

1.7 Healthy Eating

Those in favour of genetically modified vegetables will argue that organic farming does use pesticide. This is true especially when pest populations get out of balance. Growers are then encouraged to try various options like insect predators, mating disruption, traps, and barriers. If these fail, permission may be granted by the certifier to apply botanical or other non-persistent pest controls under restricted conditions. However, genetically modified produce requires at least 26 per cent more pesticide per acre. Not enough awareness has been raised about this and customers do not know the disadvantages of this.

This was recently highlighted when Monsanto lost a civil suit against them by French farmer, Paul Francois, on 23 February 2012. The farmer claimed that since being exposed to Monsanto's Lasso in 2004, he had developed severe neurological problems such as memory loss and headaches. This same pesticide was banned by some countries in the European Union in 2007 and the recent victory of Francois was able to raise awareness for others who are facing similar issues.

Some organisations insist that Parkinson's also stems from severe and prolonged pesticide poisoning but medical researchers have not accepted this. The nasty side effects of pesticide do not stop at the farmer; it often transfers to the plants, soil, animals that eat the grass and eventually those who eat the infected meat and vegetables. While it can be argued that this is an exaggerated version of how contamination can break the food chain, one must always remember that such contamination is often permanent or take a long time to fix.

Chief Scientist of the Oregon Organic Centre, Dr Charles Benbrook stated that, "Organic farmers do not use toxic synthetic pesticides, hormones to hasten animal growth and increase production, genetic modification or genetically modified feed, or artificial fertilizers. Instead, they use management practices that restore, maintain, and enhance soil health and ecosystem integrity."

Pioneer environmentalist and founder of the Soil Association, Lady Eve Balfour has stressed that the criteria for a sustainable agriculture is dependent on permanence. This would mean that farmers would have to adopt techniques that maintain soil fertility indefinitely and they would have to utilise only renewable sources as much as they can. Farmers also need to make a conscious effort to not grossly pollute the environment, and to foster biological activity within the soil and throughout the cycles of all the involved food chains.

Waitrose has demonstrated for this statement and agrees that organic farming and all organic farmers have to follow certain rules which impacts on the food they produce. Organic produce is cultivated using a system of crop rotation, a method that helps to keep the soil healthy. Organic agriculture aims to be sustainable and to maintain land in a healthy, fertile state for future generations. Organic growing techniques focus on maintaining a healthy soil and minimise the use of pesticides. Thus, environmental pollution is limited and wildlife protected and regenerated.

It is virtually impossible for a consumer to know of all these happenings before they eat what is on their plates. It for this simple reason, that food labels and accurate product information for meat and vegetables are necessary.

1.8 Knowledge is Power

People cannot be forced to eat produce that is genetically modified. At the very least, they must be given options. Just as they are given the option to choose between different brands, genetically modified produce must be marked clearly. How will this affect Monsanto and other companies that produce these products?

Take for example the Flavr Savr tomato, which was the first genetically engineered crop product to be commercialised. Authors G. Bruening and J.M. Lyons stated in a research paper, "The research and marketing efforts that produced the FLAVR SAVR tomato resulted in scientific success, a temporary sales success, and then commercial demise. The FLAVR SAVR story reveals how difficult it can be to bring genetically engineered products to market, how objections with little or no scientific merit can influence the outcome, and how important public opinion is in determining commercial success."

In 2001, Monsanto was forced to recall 10 per cent of its genetically modified canola seed after trace amounts of herbicide were found in it. While the company argued that the recall stemmed from a regulatory issue and was not a health issue, Canadian Health Officials called for more guidelines on genetically modified produce. In 2009, an appeals court in the United States upheld a previous ruling that banned Monsanto from selling its genetically modified RoundUp Ready Alfafa. Research indicated that the use of the company's pesticide Round Up was prevalent and was not safe for human consumption.

Aside from the issue of recognising genetically modified produce, awareness should also be raised about its carbon footprint. Consumers should be able to recognise which products are more damaging to the environment. At this stage, most buy fresh and processed food without realising they are actually harming their own environment. In March 2010, the UK Government requested that all supermarket food labels indicate country of origin, animal welfare standards and carbon footprint. Some of the first few companies to volunteer their support were Asda, Tesco's and Sainsbury's.

If this effort can be extended to products outside food labels, and electrical goods were also able to have a carbon footprint label, consumers would definitely be more aware and cautious of their purchases. Computer giant, Apple Inc. has made significant progress in informing consumers about its carbon footprint by posting regular updates on its "green" initiatives on its website and by reducing its packaging sizes by at least 42 per cent.

Why is carbon footprint important and how does it even affect the food chain? Food miles play a crucial point to the connection of both. In other words, how much distance food takes to get to your plate determines its impact on the environment. While a particular food item may not be available throughout the year, and food miles may increase because of seasonality, it is long-term sustainability that suffers in the end and permanently altering the food chain. Additionally, carbon emissions used when packaging and storing red meat are significantly higher than other types of food.

If communities were encouraged to eat locally and more awareness was raised on the issue of food miles, there is a strong chance demand can be altered and the carbon footprint lowered. Again, this is a long-term strategy and its results may not be felt in the beginning.

1.9 Combined Efforts

Albert Einstein said "We can't solve problems by using the same kind of thinking we used when we created them." While he was not referring to sustainability at the time, it is an apt quote that describes the debate of sustainable living. In decades to come, the fear of not having enough food for the world population stems from the current rush to maximize nature's resources.

In the long-term, this has resulted in climate change, limited resources and unstable economies around the globe. Genetically modified produce looks tempting as an option but it is a short-term resolve and one that will cause more damage to soil. Organic farming appears challenging and may not always produce the desired quantity but it is able to sustain a healthier community.

However, sustainable living cannot and will not be achieved by one large effort alone, no matter the amount of money that is spent on it. There have to be combined efforts from different governments and different levels of society.

For example, employees at Johnson Matthey's Massachusetts's branch actively pursued 43 different sustainable options in April 2008. Paper and plastic kitchenware were replaced with reusable ones and a reusable bag was designed for employees to use instead of paper and plastic bags. Seminars were given and feedback was sought on other methods the company needed to take to ensure it was reducing energy and its employees understood the impact of waste management.

These are no longer new measures as more schools and offices carry out these awareness programmes. Grocery merchants around the world have asked for their customers to bring their own bags or no longer hand out plastic bags anymore.

Environmental awareness programmes such as the Earth Summit and Earth Hour have become increasingly popular. Earth Hour started in Sydney in 2006 when the local World Wildlife Fund asked for support towards climate change action. In 2007, more than 2.2 million locals supported this campaign by turning their lights out for one hour. In the following years, the event became global and is scheduled every year on the last Saturday of every March.

In 2011, hundreds of millions of people from at least 135 countries participated in the event which called for an extension of the programme; it called for people to go beyond one-hour conservation to long-term conservation. Younger members of communities are starting to see the importance of recycling and conservation.

The 2012 Earth Summit is focused on education as a means of awareness for the issue of sustainability. However, alongside educating the public, the summit also needs to address issues such as pollution and mismanagement of natural resources before they occur. As with other things in life, prevention is better than cure. Alternatively, steps towards fixing these mishaps need to be enforced more stringently. For instance, the oil spill that occurred in the Gulf of Mexico in April 2010 has affected at least 6,500 kilometres to 180,000 kilometres of land and sea. Dolphins, whales and other sea life are dying twice as regularly as when the spill occurred and oil residue on the seabed was not degrading when discovered in February 2011. While the disaster itself may not have been preventable, conservation efforts should receive more funding and awareness to ensure limited interruption to the food chain.

All of this seems to be out of topic when thinking about genetically modified produce but if conservation efforts are made, and sustainability becomes a must in every home, will genetically modified produce be a necessity?

1.10 Conclusion

Sustainability isn't a recent debate and it probably will go on for at a few more decades. The choice between comfort and ensuring sustaining resources appears to be one that many will not choose. However, as much as the discussion of these points highlighted moderation, it also proves that genetically modified produce is not the only solution towards achieving sustainability.

Sustainable living is not a single nation's problem. It is everyone's problem and the sooner it is dealt with the better.

Opinion Poll - But What Are You Eating

An opinion poll (*But What Are You Eating*) was conducted from 15th February 2012 to 5th March 2012. The poll targeted at least 37 different people from various countries, locations and occupations who were invited to share their thoughts on this topic.

1. Are you aware that genetically modified fruits and vegetables exist?

Yes – 34 participants

No – 3 participants

2. It is argued, that genetically modified fruits and vegetables are needed to ensure there is long-term food supply. Do you agree with this?

Yes – 8 participants

No – 24 participants

Don't know – 1 participant

More information required – 4 participants

3. Which would you choose to ensure sustainability?
Genetically modified fruits and vegetables – 5 participants
Organic farming – 25 participants
Both – 5 participants
Permaculture – 1
Responsible farming and land management – 1

4. If genetically modified fruit and vegetables were being sold in your local store, would you want to know the side effects?
Yes – 33 participants
No – 4 participants

DEMOGRAPHICS OF PARTICIPANTS

1. Location
USA – 26 participants
United Kingdom – 7 participants
India – 3 participants
Phillipines – 1 participant

2. Age
18 to 25 – 7 participants
26 to 35 – 8 participants
36 to 45 – 7 participants
46 to 55 – 9 participants
56 and above – 6 participants

3. Gender
Femle – 29 participants
Male – 8 participants

Participants were also invited to share their opinions and thoughts on the subject matter. Some of the responses that were recorded are indicated below.

1. Eating GM foods is probably safe. It's the effect of such crops on the wider environment that is the worrying aspect. We know that evolution depends on tiny mutations in the genes of organisms. It seems lunatic to introduce deliberate mutation without first having a very sound knowledge of what effects these may have on future interbreeding of such modified crops with natural plants.

2. I believe genetically modified and pesticides are the main reason for autoimmune deficiencies in this country. Cooperative organic farming would allow better health and longevity. If we focused more on creating natural energy using cooperative methods we might stand a chance in the future. Everyone should have access to a garden and those who can should help those who cannot.

3. I think it is far too early to know the ramifications of using/eating GM produce - until we know more we can't rely on it for sustainability. That said, there have been remarkable interventions to food crops that have saved many lives so we can't just write GM off as 'bad'.

4. It would take extensive testing and trials to get genetically modified food ready for stores. Even if only the gene controlling speed of growth is changed, different groups of genes together have effects as well, and this food would first have to be tested on animals, then be put through extensive human trials. The people in the trials would probably have to have their own genes mapped so scientists could ensure the food was tested with all major gene variations in people.

The cost of all this would send prices for food through the roof. It costs a lot of money to train a geneticist and keep up the equipment needed for genetic modification. If this were offered as another option in addition to regular food, no one would opt to pay the price and the endeavour may fail simply for lack of funding. To replace all food with this and not give people an option, there would be fits and riots going on for the increase in price for food and there would be more poor people unable to feed themselves. This is something that would have to be introduced very slowly and carefully, and may only succeed if enough people are willing to work or fund it without making any profits.

5. Like most other things, I believe in consumers being able to make educated choices. If a consumer has easy access to both the risks and benefits of ANY sort of food choices, then they should be allowed to make a decision based on their own situation as to which products they buy. Clear labelling and education programs are, IMHO, what are needed most.

While I personally would choose organic methods of farming over genetically modified food, due to all of the side effects of GMO production, antibiotics/hormones, and pesticides, the cost of organic food as well as the unclear labelling of organic foods (as in, some things are allowed to be labelled as "organic" when by the strictest standards, they are not), make it an unappealing choice for many.

In addition, when thinking on a global scale, sometimes it's better to have food that could potentially cause health problems in the future (such as genetically modified produce and food derived from GMO's) than to starve, and that's a very real concern in some areas.

6. We need true data with comparisons, instead of anecdotal data that doesn't really tell us anything but isolated events. With a real, comprehensive study by the medical/scientific community can we really know if there is a problem with these foods? Like many issues, I suspect the answer is somewhere in the middle.

The world doesn't lack capacity to make food; we lack capacity to get food where it needs to be. Americans are obese while developing countries starve. The farming industry is very tenuous financially to say the least and a very complex situation with no simple solutions.

About the author

Bruno McGrath graduated from the University of West London and has been a professional chef for more than ten years. He is well-known for his diversified palate and food philosophy which is focused on ensuring sustainable living while enjoying well-balanced meals.

Bibliography

Ayers, J. (2012) *300,000 Organic Farmers Sue Monsanto in Federal Court.* [online] Available from: < http://www.nationofchange.org/300000-organic-farmers-sue-monsanto-federal-court-decision-march-31st-go-trial-1329059467> [Accessed on 15th Feb 2012].

Barlett, D, L. Steele, J. (2008) *Monsanto's Harvest of Fear.* [online] Available from: < http://www.vanityfair.com/politics/features/2008/05/monsanto200805> [Accessed on 15th Feb 2012].

BBC News. (2011) *Eurozone seeks bailout funds from China.* [online] Available from: < http://www.bbc.co.uk/news/world-europe-15489202> [Accessed on 10th Feb 2012].

Benbrook, Dr, C. (2009) *Impacts of Genetically Engineered Crops on Pesticide Use: The First Thirteen Years.* [online] Available from: < http://www.organic-center.org/science.pest.php?action=view&report_id=159> [Accessed on 10th Feb 2012].

Benbrook, Dr, C. (2008) *Prevention, not Profit, should Drive Pest Management.* [online] Available from: < http://www.organic-center.org/organic101.html> [Accessed on 11th Feb 2012].

Bruening, G. Lyons, J, M. (2000) *The case of the FLAVR SAVR tomato.* [online] Available from < http://ucanr.org/repository/cao/landingpage.cfm?article=ca.v054n04p6&fulltext=yes> [Accessed on 9th Feb 2012].

Chinese Embassy. (2011) *Family Planning in China.* [online] Available from: < http://www.fmprc.gov.cn/ce/celt/eng/zt/zfbps/t125241.htm> [Accessed on 12th Feb 2012].

Coca Cola. (2012) *Refrigeration.* [online] Available from: < http://www.thecoca-colacompany.com/citizenship/refrigeration_equipment.html> [Accessed on 13th Feb 2012].

Confino, J. (2010) *Should the media be more supportive of cor-*

porate moves towards sustainability? [online] Available from: < http://www.guardian.co.uk/sustainability/blog/7> [Accessed on 17th Feb 2012].

Engelman, R. (2009) *Population and Sustainability: Can We Avoid Limiting the Number of People?* [online] Available from: < http://www.scientificamerican.com/article.cfm?id=population-and-sustainability> [Accessed on 18th Feb 2012].

Foskett, D. Ceserani, V. (2007) *The Theory of Catering*. 11th ed. London: Hodder Arnold.

Greenpeace. (2000) *Incidents where genetic engineering has gone wrong.* [online] Available from: < http://archive.greenpeace.org/comms/97/geneng/getoogoo.html#Case> [Accessed on 20th Feb 2012].

Heasman, M. Lang, T. (2004) *Food Wars. The Battle for Mouths, Minds and Markets*. London: Earthscan Ltd.

Huffington Post. (2012) *Heston Blumenthal's £207,000 Test Tube Burger Is First Beef Patty Created In A Lab.* [online] Available from: < http://www.huffingtonpost.co.uk/2012/02/20/heston-blumenthals-207000-test-tube-burger-is-first-beef-patty-created-in-a-lab_n_1288365.html> [Accessed on 22nd Feb 2012].

IFOAM, (2012) *Genetic Engineering vs. Organic Farming.* [online] Available from: < http://www.ifoam.org/growing_organic/1_arguments_for_oa/environmental_benefits/ge_vs_oa.html> [Accessed on 1st March 2012].

Monsanto. (2012) *Monsanto in the News.* [online] Available from: < http://www.monsanto.com/newsviews/Pages/default.aspx> [Accessed on 18th Feb 2012].

Patel, R. (2008) *Stuffed and Starved. Markets, Power and the Hidden Battle for the World Food System*. London: Portobello Books Ltd.

Permaculture Institute. (2012) *Permacuture – Key Concepts.* [online] Available from: < http://www.permaculture.org/nm/

index.php/site/key_concepts> [Accessed on 15th Feb 2012].

Pfeiffer, A. (2006) *Eating Fossil Fuels: Oil, Food and the Coming Crisis in Agriculture*. Canada: New Society Publishers.

Subramaniam, A. (2011) *Organic Farming or Genetic Engineering?* [online] Available from: < http://www.study-in.de/en/community/tandem-reporters/--16453> [Accessed on 18th Feb 2012].

Telford, R. (2012) *Permaculture Principles*. [online] Available from: < http://permacultureprinciples.com/contact.php#davidholmgren> [Accessed on 11th Feb 2012].

UNCSD. (2012) *Objective & Themes*. [online] Available from: < http://www.uncsd2012.org/rio20/objectiveandthemes.html> [Accessed on 15th Feb 2012].

United Nations. (2009) *Integrated planning and management of land resources*. [online] Available from: < https://www.un.org/esa/dsd/susdevtopics/sdt_land.shtml> [Accessed on 10th Jan 2012].

Wilcox, C. (2011) *Mythbusting 101: Organic Farming > Conventional Agriculture*. [online] Available from: < http://blogs.scientificamerican.com/science-sushi/2011/07/18/mythbusting-101-organic-farming-conventional-agriculture/> [Accessed on 16th Feb 2012].

Made in the USA
Lexington, KY
16 May 2014